The Vibrant Diabetic Diet Cooking Book for Beginners

Lose Weight and Surprise Your Friends with Effortless and Healthy Recipes

Lesly Mclean

Table of contents

WARM AVO AND QUINOA SALAD 6

TUNA SALAD 8

HERRING & VEGGIES SOUP 10

SALMON SOUP 13

SALMON & SHRIMP STEW 15

SALMON CURRY 18

SALMON WITH BELL PEPPERS 21

SHRIMP SALAD 24

SHRIMP & VEGGIES CURRY 27

SHRIMP WITH ZUCCHINI 30

SHRIMP WITH BROCCOLI 32

PORK CHOP DIANE...34

AUTUMN PORK CHOPS WITH RED CABBAGE AND APPLES 37

FLOURLESS CHOCOLATE CAKE 40

RASPBERRY CAKE WITH WHITE CHOCOLATE SAUCE 43

KETOGENIC LAVA CAKE..46

KETOGENIC CHEESE CAKE 48

CAKE WITH WHIPPED CREAM ICING 51

WALNUT-FRUIT CAKE 54

GINGER CAKE..57

KETOGENIC ORANGE CAKE 60

LEMON CAKE 63

ROASTED CUMIN CARROTS 66

TASTY & TENDER BRUSSELS SPROUTS 68

SAUTÉED VEGGIES 70

MUSTARD GREEN BEANS..72

ZUCCHINI FRIES 74

BROCCOLI NUGGETS..76

ZUCCHINI CAULIFLOWER FRITTERS 78

ROASTED CHICKPEAS..80

PEANUT BUTTER MOUSSE 82

COFFEE MOUSSE...84

WILD RICE AND BLACK LENTILS BOWL 86

ALKALINE SPAGHETTI SQUASH RECIPE 90

DAIRY-FREE FRUIT TARTS 92

SPAGHETTI SQUASH WITH PEANUT SAUCE 94

CAULIFLOWER ALFREDO PASTA..97

SLOPPY JOE 100

AMARETTI 103

GREEN FRUIT JUICE...105

KALE CHICKPEA MASH 107

QUINOA AND APPLE..109

4

Warm Avo And Quinoa Salad

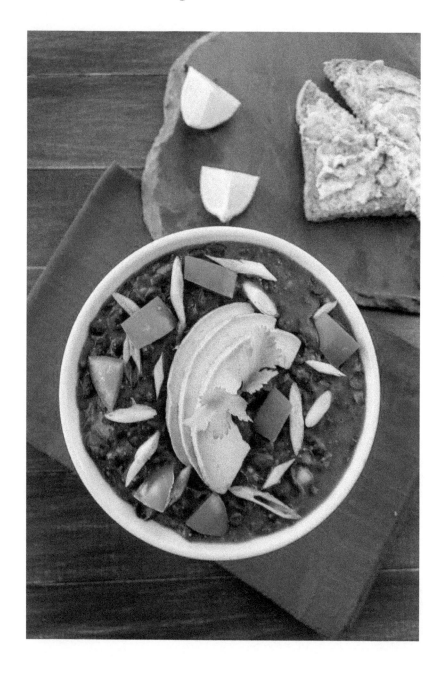

This is an amazing alkaline quinoa dish that will blow your mind away. It's an easy dish that will be ready in less than 20 minutes.

Preparation Time : 5 minutes

Cooking Time : 12 minutes

Servings : 4

Ingredients :

- 4 ripe avocados, quartered

- 1 cup quinoa

- 0.9 lb. Chickpeas, drained

- 1 oz flat leaf parsley

Directions :

1. Add quinoa in a pot with 2 cups of water. Bring to boil then simmer for 12 minutes or until all the water has evaporated. The grains should be glassy and swollen.

2. Toss the quinoa with all other Ingredients and season with salt and pepper to taste.

3. Serve with olive oil and lemon wedges. Enjoy.

Nutrition : Calories: 354; Total fat: 16 g; Saturated fat: 2 g; Net Carbs: 31 g; Protein: 15 g; Sugars: 6 g; Fiber: 15 g; Sodium: 226 mg; Potassium: 205 mg

Tuna Salad

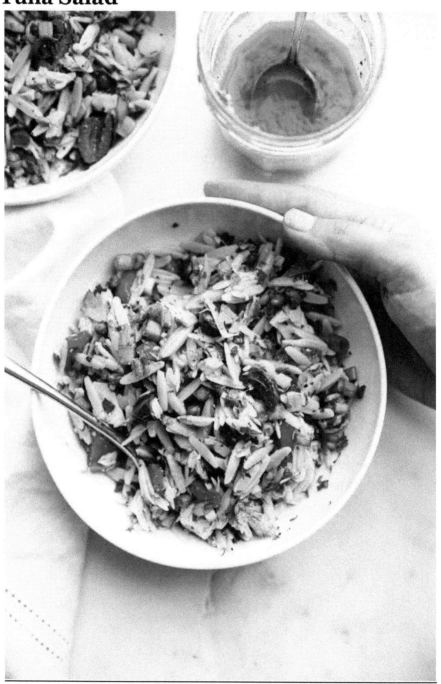

Preparation Time : 15 minutes

Cooking Time : 30 minutes

Servings : 2

Ingredients :

- 2 (5-ounce) cans water packed tuna, drained
- 2 tablespoons fat-free plain Greek yogurt
- Salt and ground black pepper, as required
- 2 medium carrots, peeled and shredded
- 2 apples, cored and chopped
- 2 cups fresh spinach, torn

Directions :

1. In a large bowl, add the tuna, yogurt, salt and black pepper and gently, stir to combine.
2. Add the carrots and apples and stir to combine.
3. Serve immediately.

Nutrition : Calories 306; Total Fat 1.8g; Saturated Fat 0 g; Cholesterol 63 mg; Total Carbs 38 g; Sugar 26 g; Fiber 7.6 g; Sodium 324 mg; Potassium 602 mg; Protein 35.8 g

Herring & Veggies Soup

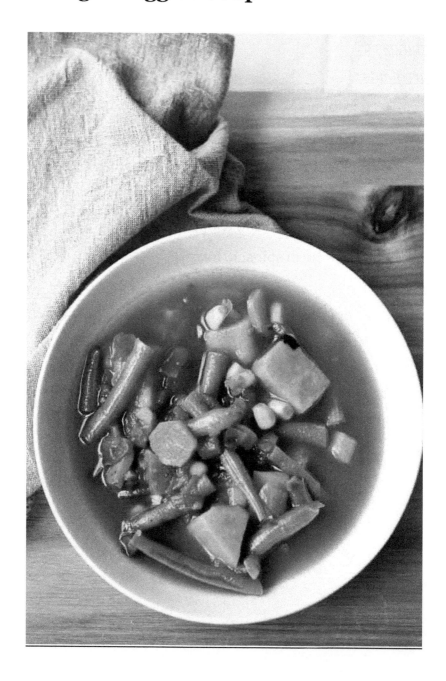

Preparation Time : 15 minutes

Cooking Time : 25 minutes

Servings : 5

Ingredients :

- 2 tablespoons olive oil
- 1 shallot, chopped
- 2 small garlic cloves, minced
- 1 jalapeño pepper, chopped
- 1 head cabbage, chopped
- 1 small red bell pepper, seeded and chopped finely
- 1 small yellow bell pepper, seeded and chopped finely
- 5 cups low-sodium chicken broth
- 2 (4-ounce) boneless herring fillets, cubed
- ¼ cup fresh cilantro, minced
- 2 tablespoons fresh lemon juice
- Ground black pepper, as required
- 2 scallions, chopped

Directions :

1. In a large soup pan, heat the oil over medium heat and sauté shallot and garlic for 2-3 minutes.
2. Add the cabbage and bell peppers and sauté for about 3-4 minutes.
3. Add the broth and bring to a boil over high heat.
4. Now, reduce the heat to medium-low and simmer for about 10 minutes.

5. Add the herring cubes and cook for about 5-6 minutes.

6. Stir in the cilantro, lemon juice, salt and black pepper and cook for about 1-2 minutes.

7. Serve hot with the topping of scallion.

Nutrition : Calories 215; Total Fat 11.2g; Saturated Fat 2.1 g; Cholesterol 35 mg; Total Carbs 14.7 g; Sugar 7 g; Fiber 4.5 g; Sodium 152 mg; Potassium 574 mg; Protein 15.1 g

Salmon Soup

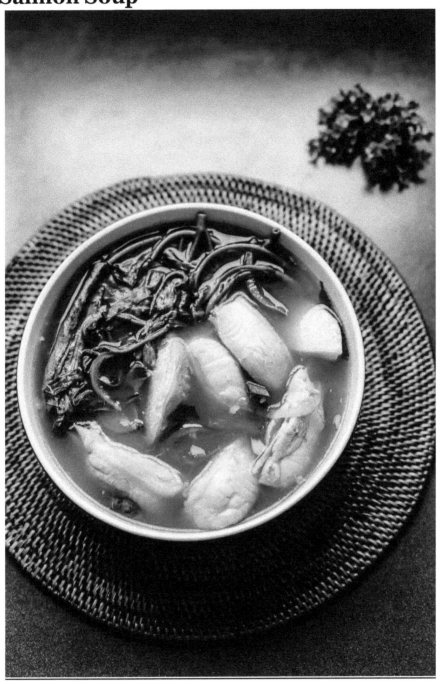

Preparation Time : 15 minutes

Cooking Time : 20 minutes

Servings : 4

Ingredients :

- 1 tablespoon olive oil
- 1 yellow onion, chopped
- 1 garlic clove, minced
- 4 cups low-sodium chicken broth
- 1-pound boneless salmon, cubed
- 2 tablespoon fresh cilantro, chopped
- Ground black pepper, as required
- 1 tablespoon fresh lime juice

Directions :

1. In a large pan heat the oil over medium heat and sauté the onion for about 5 minutes.
2. Add the garlic and sauté for about 1 minute.
3. Stir in the broth and bring to a boil over high heat.
4. Now, reduce the heat to low and simmer for about 10 minutes.
5. Add the salmon and soy sauce and cook for about 3-4 minutes.
6. Stir in black pepper, lime juice, and cilantro and serve hot.

Nutrition : Calories 208; Total Fat 10.5 g; Saturated Fat 1.5 g; Cholesterol 50 mg; Total Carbs 3.9 g; Sugar 1.2 g; Fiber 0.6 g; Sodium 121 mg; Potassium 331 mg; Protein 24.4 g

Salmon & Shrimp Stew

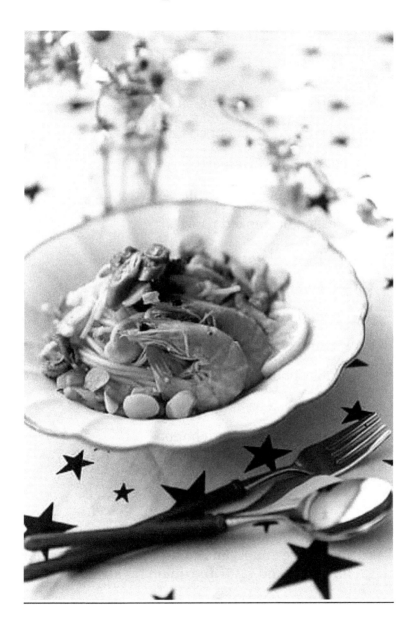

Preparation Time : 20 minutes

Cooking Time : 21 minutes

Servings : 6

Ingredients :

- 2 tablespoons olive oil
- 1/2 cup onion, chopped finely
- 2 garlic cloves, minced
- 1 Serrano pepper, chopped
- 1 teaspoon smoked paprika
- 4 cups fresh tomatoes, chopped
- 4 cups low-sodium chicken broth
- 1 pound salmon fillets, cubed
- 1 pound shrimp, peeled and deveined
- 2 tablespoons fresh lime juice
- ¼ cup fresh basil, chopped
- ¼ cup fresh parsley, chopped
- Ground black pepper, as required
- 2 scallions, chopped

Directions :

1. In a large soup pan, melt coconut oil over medium-high heat and sauté the onion for about 5-6 minutes.

2. Add the garlic, Serrano pepper and smoked paprika and sauté for about 1 minute.

3. Add the tomatoes and broth and bring to a gentle simmer over medium heat.

4. Simmer for about 5 minutes.

5. Add the salmon and simmer for about 3-4 minutes.

6. Stir in the remaining seafood and cook for about 4-5 minutes.

7. Stir in the lemon juice, basil, parsley, sea salt and black pepper and remove from heat.

8. Serve hot with the garnishing of scallion.

Nutrition : Calories 271; Total Fat 11 g; Saturated Fat 1.8 g; Cholesterol 193 mg; Total Carbs 8.6 g; Sugar 3.8 g; Fiber 2.1 g; Sodium 273 mg; Potassium 763 mg; Protein 34.7 g

Salmon Curry

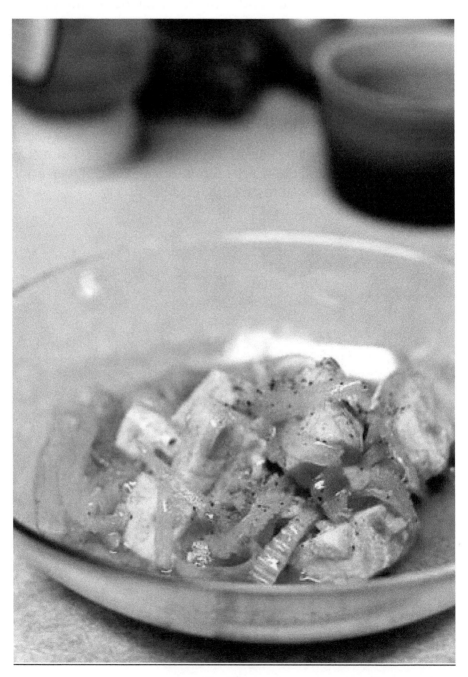

Preparation Time : 15 minutes

Cooking Time : 30 minutes

Servings : 6

Ingredients :

- 6 (4-ounce) salmon fillets
- 1 teaspoon ground turmeric, divided
- Salt, as required
- 3 tablespoon olive oil, divided
- 1 yellow onion, chopped finely
- 1 teaspoon garlic paste
- 1 teaspoon fresh ginger paste
- 3-4 green chilies, halved
- 1 teaspoon red chili powder
- 1/2 teaspoon ground cumin
- 1/2 teaspoon ground cinnamon
- ¾ cup fat-free plain Greek yogurt, whipped
- ¾ cup filtered water
- 3 tablespoon fresh cilantro, chopped

Directions :

1. Season each salmon fillet with 1/2 teaspoon of the turmeric and salt.

2. In a large skillet, melt 1 tablespoon of the butter over medium heat and cook the salmon fillets for about 2 minutes per side.

3. Transfer the salmon onto a plate.

4. In the same skillet, melt the remaining butter over medium heat and sauté the onion for about 4-5 minutes.

5. Add the garlic paste, ginger paste, green chilies, remaining turmeric and spices and sauté for about 1 minute.

6. Now, reduce the heat to medium-low.

7. Slowly, add the yogurt and water, stirring continuously until smooth.

8. Cover the skillet and simmer for about 10-15 minutes or until desired doneness of the sauce.

9. Carefully, add the salmon fillets and simmer for about 5 minutes.

10. Serve hot with the garnishing of cilantro.

Nutrition : Calories 242; Total Fat 14.3 g; Saturated Fat 2 g; Cholesterol 51 mg; Total Carbs 4.1 g; Sugar 2 g; Fiber 0.8 g; Sodium 98 mg; Potassium 493 mg; Protein 25.4 g

Salmon with Bell Peppers

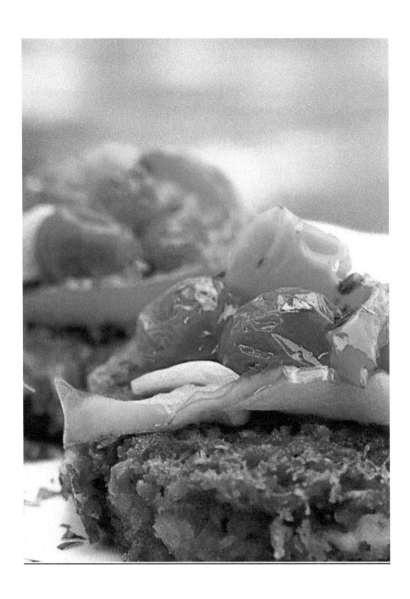

Preparation Time : 15 minutes

Cooking Time : 20 minutes

Servings : 6

Ingredients :

- 6 (3-ounce) salmon fillets
- Pinch of salt
- Ground black pepper, as required
- 1 yellow bell pepper, seeded and cubed
- 1 red bell pepper, seeded and cubed
- 4 plum tomatoes, cubed
- 1 small onion, sliced thinly
- 1/2 cup fresh parsley, chopped
- ¼ cup olive oil
- 2 tablespoons fresh lemon juice

Directions :

1. Preheat the oven to 400 degrees F.
2. Season each salmon fillet with salt and black pepper lightly.
3. In a bowl, mix together the bell peppers, tomato and onion.
4. Arrange 6 foil pieces onto a smooth surface.
5. Place 1 salmon fillet over each foil paper and sprinkle with salt and black pepper.

6. Place veggie mixture over each fillet evenly and top with parsley and capers evenly.

7. Drizzle with oil and lemon juice.

8. Fold each foil around salmon mixture to seal it.

9. Arrange the foil packets onto a large baking sheet in a single layer.

10. Bake for about 20 minutes

11. Serve hot

Nutrition : Calories 220; Total Fat 14 g; Saturated Fat 2 g; Cholesterol 38 mg; Total Carbs 7.7 g; Sugar 4.8 g; Fiber 2 g; Sodium 74 mg; Potassium 647 mg; Protein 17.9 g

Shrimp Salad

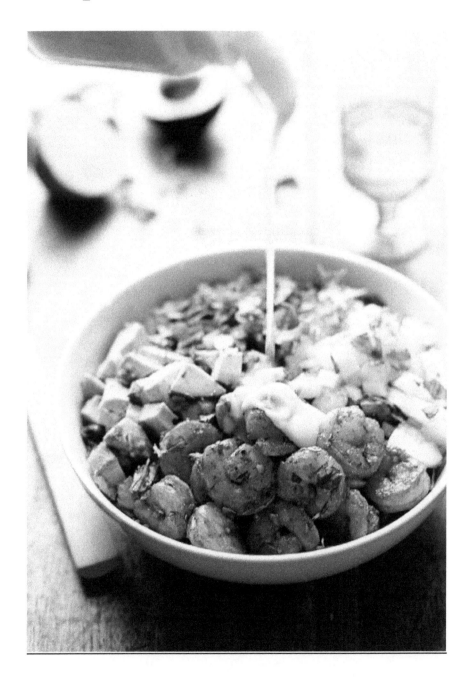

Preparation Time : 20 minutes

Cooking Time : 4 minutes

Servings : 6

Ingredients :

For Salad:

- 1 pound shrimp, peeled and deveined
- Salt and ground black pepper, as required
- 1 teaspoon olive oil
- 11/2 cups carrots, peeled and julienned
- 11/2 cups red cabbage, shredded
- 11/2 cup cucumber, julienned
- 5 cups fresh baby arugula
- ¼ cup fresh basil, chopped
- ¼ cup fresh cilantro, chopped
- 4 cups lettuce, torn
- ¼ cup almonds, chopped

For Dressing:

- 2 tablespoons natural almond butter
- 1 garlic clove, crushed
- 1 tablespoon fresh cilantro, chopped
- 1 tablespoon fresh lime juice
- 1 tablespoon unsweetened applesauce
- 2 teaspoons balsamic vinegar
- 1/2 teaspoon cayenne pepper

- Salt, as required

- 1 tablespoon water

- 1/3 cup olive oil

Directions :

1. Slowly, add the oil, beating continuously until smooth.

2. For salad: in a bowl, add shrimp, salt, black pepper and oil and toss to coat well.

3. Heat a skillet over medium-high heat and cook the shrimp for about 2 minutes per side.

4. Remove from the heat and set aside to cool.

5. In a large bowl, add the shrimp, vegetables and mix well.

6. For dressing: in a bowl, add all ingredients except oil and beat until well combined.

7. Place the dressing over shrimp mixture and gently, toss to coat well.

8. Serve immediately.

Nutrition : Calories 274; Total Fat 17.7 g; Saturated Fat 2.4 g; Cholesterol 159 mg; Total Carbs 10 g; Sugar 3.8 g; Fiber 2.9 g; Sodium 242 mg; Potassium 481 mg; Protein 20.5 g

Shrimp & Veggies Curry

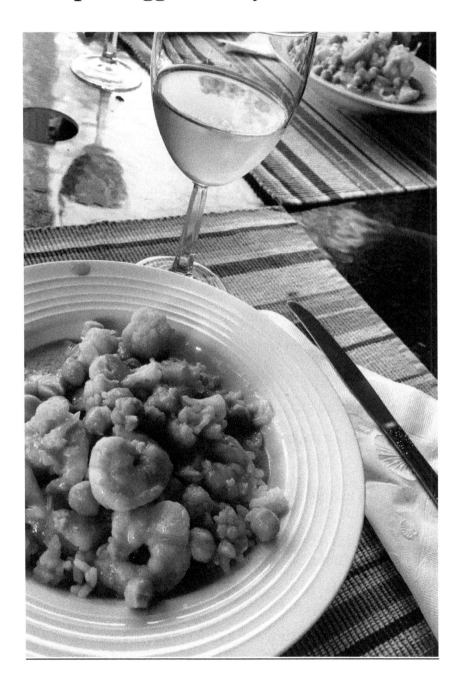

Preparation Time : 20 minutes

Cooking Time : 20 minutes

Servings : 6

Ingredients :

- 2 teaspoons olive oil
- 11/2 medium white onions, sliced
- 2 medium green bell peppers, seeded and sliced
- 3 medium carrots, peeled and sliced thinly
- 3 garlic cloves, chopped finely
- 1 tablespoon fresh ginger, chopped finely
- 21/2 teaspoons curry powder
- 11/2 pounds shrimp, peeled and deveined
- 1 cup filtered water
- 2 tablespoons fresh lime juice
- Salt and ground black pepper, as required
- 2 tablespoons fresh cilantro, chopped

Directions :

1. In a large skillet, heat oil over medium-high heat and sauté the onion for about 4-5 minutes.

2. Add the bell peppers and carrot and sauté for about 3-4 minutes.

3. Add the garlic, ginger and curry powder and sauté for about 1 minute.

4. Add the shrimp and sauté for about 1 minute.

5. Stir in the water and cook for about 4-6 minutes, stirring occasionally.

6. Stir in lime juice and remove from heat.

7. Serve hot with the garnishing of cilantro.

Nutrition : Calories 193; Total Fat 3.8 g; Saturated Fat 0.9 g; Cholesterol 239 mg; Total Carbs 12 g; Sugar 4.7 g; Fiber 2.3 g; Sodium 328 mg; Potassium 437 mg; Protein 27.1 g

Shrimp with Zucchini

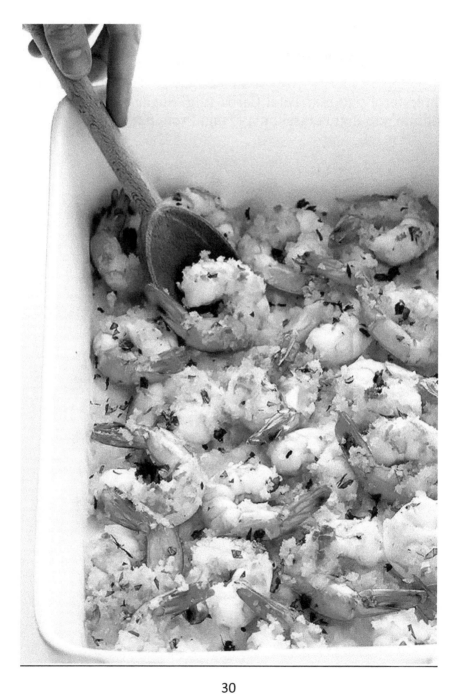

Preparation Time : 20 minutes

Cooking Time : 8 minutes

Servings : 4

Ingredients :

- 3 tablespoons olive oil
- 1-pound medium shrimp, peeled and deveined
- 1 shallot, minced
- 4 garlic cloves, minced
- ¼ teaspoon red pepper flakes, crushed
- Salt and ground black pepper, as required
- ¼ cup low-sodium chicken broth
- 2 tablespoons fresh lemon juice
- 1 teaspoon fresh lemon zest, grated finely
- 1/2-pound zucchini, spiralized with Blade C

Directions :

1. In a large skillet, heat the oil and butter over medium-high heat and cook the shrimp, shallot, garlic, red pepper flakes, salt and black pepper for about 2 minutes, stirring occasionally.

2. Stir in the broth, lemon juice and lemon zest and bring to a gentle boil.

3. Stir in zucchini noodles and cook for about 1-2 minutes.

4. Serve hot.

Nutrition : Calories 245; Total Fat 12.6 g; Saturated Fat 2.2 g; Cholesterol 239 mg; Total Carbs 5.8 g; Sugar 1.2 g; Fiber 08 g; Sodium 289 mg; Potassium 381 mg; Protein 27 g

Shrimp with Broccoli

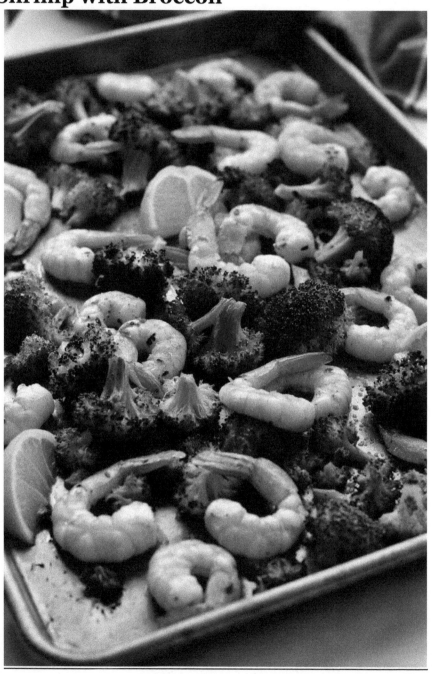

Preparation Time : 15 minutes

Cooking Time : 12 minutes

Servings : 6

Ingredients :

- 2 tablespoons olive oil, divided
- 4 cups broccoli, chopped
- 2-3 tablespoons filtered water
- 11/2 pounds large shrimp, peeled and deveined
- 2 garlic cloves, minced
- 1 (1-inch) piece fresh ginger, minced
- Salt and ground black pepper, as required

Directions :

1. In a large skillet, heat 1 tablespoon of oil over medium-high heat and cook the broccoli for about 1-2 minutes stirring continuously.

2. Stir in the water and cook, covered for about 3-4 minutes, stirring occasionally.

3. With a spoon, push the broccoli to side of the pan.

4. Add the remaining oil and let it heat.

5. Add the shrimp and cook for about 1-2 minutes, tossing occasionally.

6. Add the remaining ingredients and sauté for about 2-3 minutes.

7. Serve hot.

Nutrition : Calories 197; Total Fat 6.8 g; Saturated Fat 1.3 g; Cholesterol 239 mg; Total Carbs 6.1 g; Sugar 1.1 g; Fiber 1.6 g; Sodium 324 mg; Potassium 389 mg; Protein 27.6 g

Pork Chop Diane

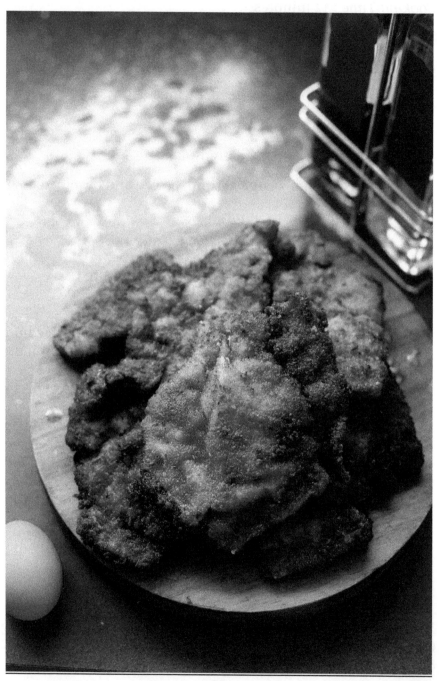

Preparation Time : 10 minutes

Cooking Time : 20 minutes

Serving : 4

Ingredients :

- ¼ cup low-sodium chicken broth
- 1 tablespoon freshly squeezed lemon juice
- 2 teaspoons Worcestershire sauce
- 2 teaspoons Dijon mustard
- 4 (5-ounce) boneless pork top loin chops
- 1 teaspoon extra-virgin olive oil
- 1 teaspoon lemon zest
- 1 teaspoon butter
- 2 teaspoons chopped fresh chives

Directions :

1. Blend together the chicken broth, lemon juice, Worcestershire sauce, and Dijon mustard and set it aside.
2. Season the pork chops lightly.
3. Situate large skillet over medium-high heat and add the olive oil.
4. Cook the pork chops, turning once, until they are no longer pink, about 8 minutes per side.
5. Put aside the chops.
6. Pour the broth mixture into the skillet and cook until warmed through and thickened, about 2 minutes.
7. Blend lemon zest, butter, and chives.

8. Garnish with a generous spoonful of sauce.

Nutrition : 200 Calories; 8g Fat; 1g Carbohydrates

Autumn Pork Chops with Red Cabbage and Apples

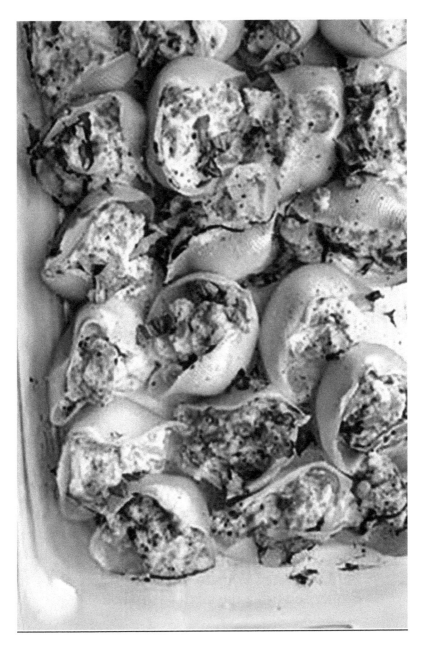

Preparation Time : 15 minutes

Cooking Time : 30 minutes

Serving : 4

Ingredients :

- ¼ cup apple cider vinegar
- 2 tablespoons granulated sweetener
- 4 (4-ounce) pork chops, about 1 inch thick
- 1 tablespoon extra-virgin olive oil
- ½ red cabbage, finely shredded
- 1 sweet onion, thinly sliced
- 1 apple, peeled, cored, and sliced
- 1 teaspoon chopped fresh thyme

Directions :

1. Scourge together the vinegar and sweetener. Set it aside.
2. Season the pork with salt and pepper.
3. Position huge skillet over medium-high heat and add the olive oil.
4. Cook the pork chops until no longer pink, turning once, about 8 minutes per side.
5. Put chops aside.
6. Add the cabbage and onion to the skillet and sauté until the vegetables have softened, about 5 minutes.
7. Add the vinegar mixture and the apple slices to the skillet and bring the mixture to a boil.

8. Adjust heat to low and simmer, covered, for 5 additional minutes.

9. Return the pork chops to the skillet, along with any accumulated juices and thyme, cover, and cook for 5 more minutes.

Nutrition : 223 Calories; 12g Carbohydrates; 3g Fiber

Flourless Chocolate Cake

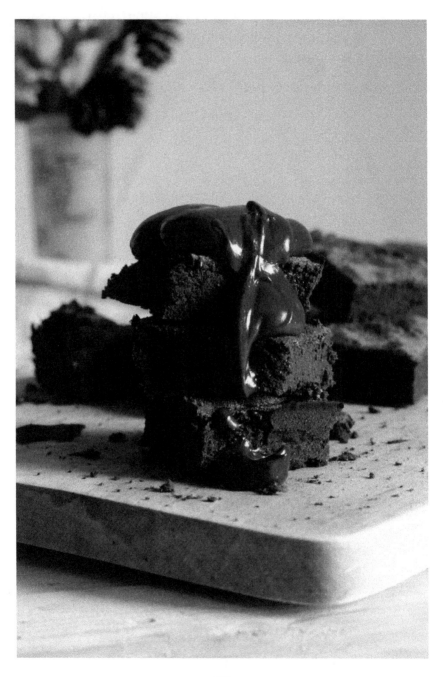

Preparation Time : 10 minutes

Cooking Time : 45 minutes

Servings : 6

Ingredients :

- 1/2 Cup of stevia
- 12 Ounces of unsweetened baking chocolate
- 2/3 Cup of ghee
- 1/3 Cup of warm water
- ¼ Teaspoon of salt
- 4 Large pastured eggs
- 2 Cups of boiling water

Directions :

1. Line the bottom of a 9-inch pan of a spring form with a parchment paper.

2. Heat the water in a small pot; then add the salt and the stevia over the water until wait until the mixture becomes completely dissolved.

3. Melt the baking chocolate into a double boiler or simply microwave it for about 30 seconds.

4. Mix the melted chocolate and the butter in a large bowl with an electric mixer.

5. Beat in your hot mixture; then crack in the egg and whisk after adding each of the eggs.

6. Pour the obtained mixture into your prepared spring form tray.

7. Wrap the spring form tray with a foil paper.

8. Place the spring form tray in a large cake tray and add boiling water right to the outside; make sure the depth doesn't exceed 1 inch.

9. Bake the cake into the water bath for about 45 minutes at a temperature of about 350 F.

10. Remove the tray from the boiling water and transfer to a wire to cool.

11. Let the cake chill for an overnight in the refrigerator.

12. Serve and enjoy your delicious cake!

Nutrition : Calories: 295; Fat: 26g; Carbohydrates: 6g; Fiber: 4g; Protein: 8g

Raspberry Cake With White Chocolate Sauce

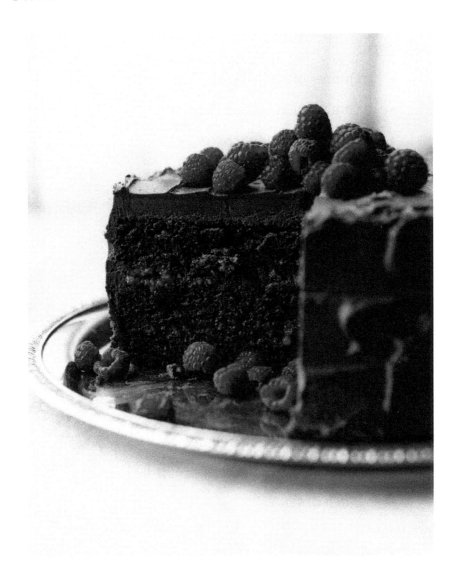

Preparation Time : 15 minutes

Cooking Time : 60 minutes

Servings : 6

Ingredients :

- 5 Ounces of melted cacao butter
- 2 Ounces of grass-fed ghee
- 1/2 Cup of coconut cream
- 1 Cup of green banana flour
- 3 Teaspoons of pure vanilla
- 4 Large eggs
- 1/2 Cup of as Lakanto Monk Fruit
- 1 Teaspoon of baking powder
- 2 Teaspoons of apple cider vinegar
- 2 Cup of raspberries

For the white chocolate sauce:

- 3 and 1/2 ounces of cacao butter
- 1/2 Cup of coconut cream
- 2 Teaspoons of pure vanilla extract
- 1 Pinch of salt

Directions :

1. Preheat your oven to a temperature of about 280 degrees Fahrenheit.

2. Combine the green banana flour with the pure vanilla extract, the baking powder, the coconut cream, the

eggs, the cider vinegar and the monk fruit and mix very well.

3. Leave the raspberries aside and line a cake loaf tin with a baking paper.

4. Pour in the batter into the baking tray and scatter the raspberries over the top of the cake.

5. Place the tray in your oven and bake it for about 60 minutes; in the meantime, prepare the sauce by

Directions for sauce:

6. Combine the cacao cream, the vanilla extract, the cacao butter and the salt in a saucepan over a low heat.

7. Mix all your ingredients with a fork to make sure the cacao butter mixes very well with the cream.

8. Remove from the heat and set aside to cool a little bit; but don't let it harden.

9. Drizzle with the chocolate sauce.

10. Scatter the cake with more raspberries.

11. Slice your cake; then serve and enjoy it!

Nutrition : Calories: 323; Fat: 31.5g; Carbohydrates: 9.9g; Fiber: 4g; Protein: 5g

Ketogenic Lava Cake

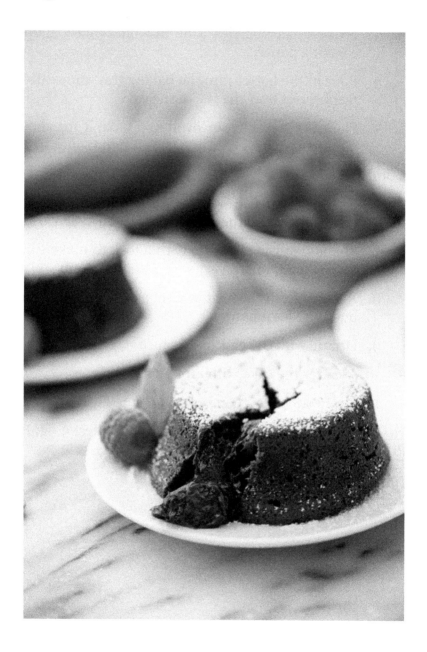

Preparation Time : 10 minutes

Cooking Time : 10 minutes

Servings : 2

Ingredients :

- 2 Oz of dark chocolate; you should at least use chocolate of 85% cocoa solids
- 1 Tablespoon of super-fine almond flour
- 2 Oz of unsalted almond butter
- 2 Large eggs

Directions :

1. Heat your oven to a temperature of about 350 Fahrenheit.
2. Grease 2 heat proof ramekins with almond butter.
3. Now, melt the chocolate and the almond butter and stir very well.
4. Beat the eggs very well with a mixer.
5. Add the eggs to the chocolate and the butter mixture and mix very well with almond flour and the swerve; then stir.
6. Pour the dough into 2 ramekins.
7. Bake for about 9 to 10 minutes.
8. Turn the cakes over plates and serve with pomegranate seeds!

Nutrition : Calories: 459; Fat: 39g; Carbohydrates: 3.5g; Fiber: 0.8g; Protein: 11.7g

Ketogenic Cheese Cake

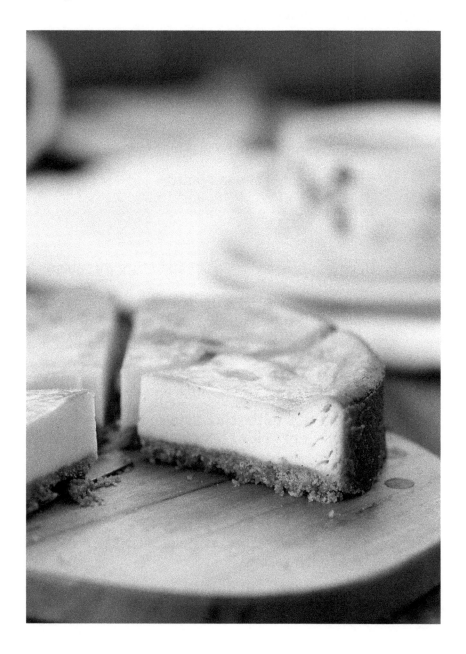

Preparation Time : 15 minutes

Cooking Time : 50 minutes

Servings : 6

Ingredients :

For the Almond Flour Cheesecake Crust:

- 2 Cups of Blanched almond flour
- 1/3 Cup of almond Butter
- 3 Tablespoons of Erythritol (powdered or granular)
- 1 Teaspoon of Vanilla extract

For the Keto Cheesecake Filling:

- 32 Oz of softened Cream cheese
- 1 and ¼ cups of powdered erythritol
- 3 Large Eggs
- 1 Tablespoon of Lemon juice
- 1 Teaspoon of Vanilla extract

Directions :

1. Preheat your oven to a temperature of about 350 degrees F.

2. Grease a spring form pan of 9¨ with cooking spray or just line its bottom with a parchment paper.

3. In order to make the cheesecake rust, stir in the melted butter, the almond flour, the vanilla extract and the erythritol in a large bowl.

4. The dough will get will be a bit crumbly; so, press it into the bottom of your prepared tray.

5. Bake for about 12 minutes; then let cool for about 10 minutes.

6. In the meantime, beat the softened cream cheese and the powdered sweetener at a low speed until it becomes smooth.

7. Crack in the eggs and beat them in at a low to medium speed until it becomes fluffy. Make sure to add one a time.

8. Add in the lemon juice and the vanilla extract and mix at a low to medium speed with a mixer.

9. Pour your filling into your pan right on top of the crust. You can use a spatula to smooth the top of the cake.

10. Bake for about 45 to 50 minutes.

11. Remove the baked cheesecake from your oven and run a knife around its edge.

12. Let the cake cool for about 4 hours in the refrigerator.

13. Serve and enjoy your delicious cheese cake!

Nutrition : Calories: 325; Fat: 29g; Carbohydrates: 6g; Fiber: 1g; Protein: 7g

Cake with Whipped Cream Icing

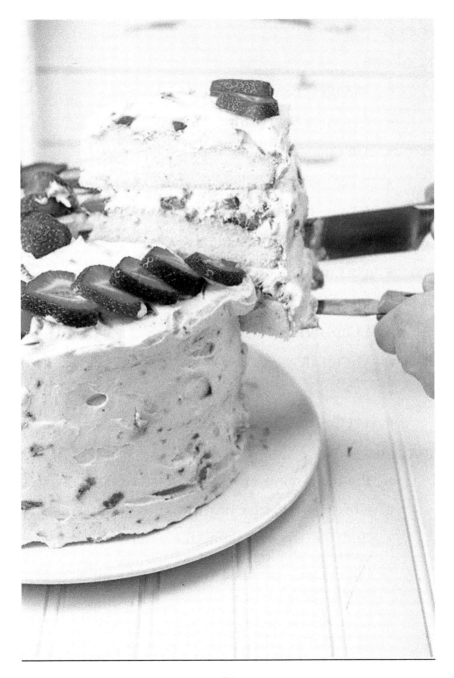

Preparation Time : 20 minutes

Cooking Time : 25 minutes

Servings : 7

Ingredients :

- ¾ Cup Coconut flour
- ¾ Cup of Swerve Sweetener
- 1/2 Cup of Cocoa powder
- 2 Teaspoons of Baking powder
- 6 Large Eggs
- 2/3 Cup of Heavy Whipping Cream
- 1/2 Cup of Melted almond Butter

For the whipped Cream Icing:

- 1 Cup of Heavy Whipping Cream
- ¼ Cup of Swerve Sweetener
- 1 Teaspoon of Vanilla extract
- 1/3 Cup of Sifted Cocoa Powder

Directions :

1. Pre-heat your oven to a temperature of about 350 F.

2. Grease an 8x8 cake tray with cooking spray.

3. Add the coconut flour, the Swerve sweetener; the cocoa powder, the baking powder, the eggs, the melted butter; and combine very well with an electric or a hand mixer.

4. Pour your batter into the cake tray and bake for about 25 minutes.

5. Remove the cake tray from the oven and let cool for about 5 minutes.

For the Icing

6. Whip the cream until it becomes fluffy; then add in the Swerve, the vanilla and the cocoa powder.

7. Add the Swerve, the vanilla and the cocoa powder; then continue mixing until your ingredients are very well combined.

8. Frost your baked cake with the icing; then slice it; serve and enjoy your delicious cake!

Nutrition : Calories: 357, Fat: 33g; Carbohydrates: 11g; Fiber: 2g; Protein: 8g

Walnut-Fruit Cake

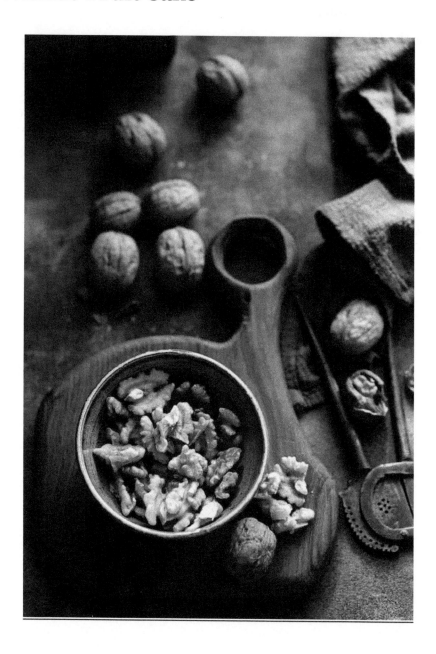

Cooking Time : 20 minutes

Servings : 6

Ingredients :

- 1/2 Cup of almond butter (softened)
- ¼ Cup of so Nourished granulated erythritol
- 1 Tablespoon of ground cinnamon
- 1/2 Teaspoon of ground nutmeg
- ¼ Teaspoon of ground cloves
- 4 Large pastured eggs
- 1 Teaspoon of vanilla extract
- 1/2 Teaspoon of almond extract
- 2 Cups of almond flour
- 1/2 Cup of chopped walnuts
- ¼ Cup of dried of unsweetened cranberries
- ¼ Cup of seedless raisins

Directions :

1. Preheat your oven to a temperature of about 350 F and grease an 8-inch baking tin of round shape with coconut oil.

2. Beat the granulated erythritol on a high speed until it becomes fluffy.

3. Add the cinnamon, the nutmeg, and the cloves; then blend your ingredients until they become smooth.

4. Crack in the eggs and beat very well by adding one at a time, plus the almond extract and the vanilla.

5. Whisk in the almond flour until it forms a smooth batter then fold in the nuts and the fruit.

6. Spread your mixture into your prepared baking pan and bake it for about 20 minutes.

7. Remove the cake from the oven and let cool for about 5 minutes.

8. Dust the cake with the powdered erythritol.

9. Serve and enjoy your cake!

Nutrition : Calories: 250; Fat: 11g; Carbohydrates: 12g; Fiber: 2g; Protein: 7g

Ginger Cake

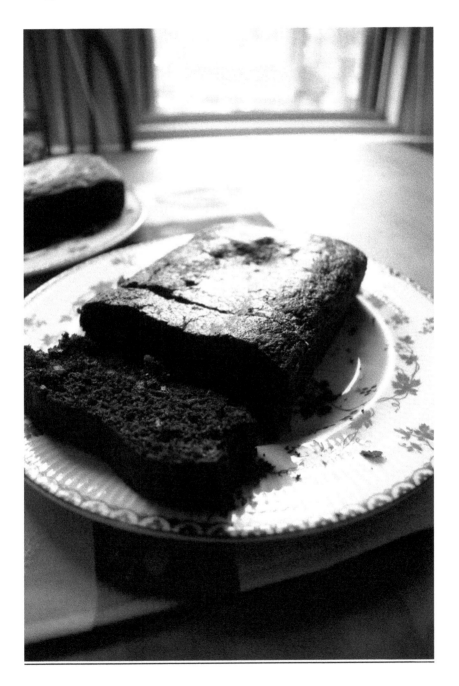

Preparation Time : 15 minutes

Cooking Time : 20 minutes

Servings : 9

Ingredients :

- 1/2 Tablespoon of unsalted almond butter to grease the pan
- 4 Large eggs
- ¼ Cup coconut milk
- 2 Tablespoons of unsalted almond butter
- 1 and 1/2 teaspoons of stevia
- 1 Tablespoon of ground cinnamon
- 1 Tablespoon of natural unweeded cocoa powder
- 1 Tablespoon of fresh ground ginger
- 1/2 Teaspoon of kosher salt
- 1 and 1/2 cups of blanched almond flour
- 1/2 Teaspoon of baking soda

Directions :

1. Preheat your oven to a temperature of 325 F.

2. Grease a glass baking tray of about 8X8 inches generously with almond butter.

3. In a large bowl, whisk all together the coconut milk, the eggs, the melted almond butter, the stevia, the cinnamon, the cocoa powder, the ginger and the kosher salt.

4. Whisk in the almond flour, then the baking soda and mix very well.

5. Pour the batter into the prepared pan and bake for about 20 to 25 minutes.

6. Let the cake cool for about 5 minutes; then slice; serve and enjoy your delicious cake.

Nutrition : Calories: 175; Fat: 15g ; Carbohydrates: 5g; Fiber: 1.9g; Protein: 5g

Ketogenic Orange Cake

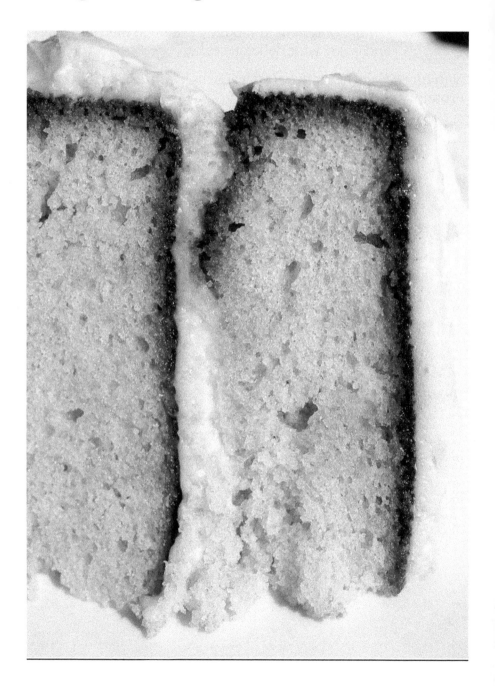

Preparation Time : 10 minutes

Cooking Time : 50minutes

Servings : 8

Ingredients :

- 2 and 1/2 cups of almond flour
- 2 Unwaxed washed oranges
- 5 Large separated eggs
- 1 Teaspoon of baking powder
- 2 Teaspoons of orange extract
- 1 Teaspoon of vanilla bean powder
- 6 Seeds of cardamom pods crushed
- 16 drops of liquid stevia; about 3 teaspoons
- 1 Handful of flaked almonds to decorate

Directions :

1. Preheat your oven to a temperature of about 350 Fahrenheit.

2. Line a rectangular bread baking tray with a parchment paper.

3. Place the oranges into a pan filled with cold water and cover it with a lid.

4. Bring the saucepan to a boil, then let simmer for about 1 hour and make sure the oranges are totally submerged.

5. Make sure the oranges are always submerged to remove any taste of bitterness.

6. Cut the oranges into halves; then remove any seeds; and drain the water and set the oranges aside to cool down.

7. Cut the oranges in half and remove any seeds, then puree it with a blender or a food processor.

8. Separate the eggs; then whisk the egg whites until you see stiff peaks forming.

9. Add all your ingredients except for the egg whites to the orange mixture and add in the egg whites; then mix.

10. Pour the batter into the cake tin and sprinkle with the flaked almonds right on top.

11. Bake your cake for about 50 minutes.

12. Remove the cake from the oven and set aside to cool for 5 minutes.

13. Slice your cake; then serve and enjoy its incredible taste!

Nutrition : Calories: 164; Fat: 12g; Carbohydrates: 7.1; Fiber: 2.7g; Protein: 10.9g

Lemon Cake

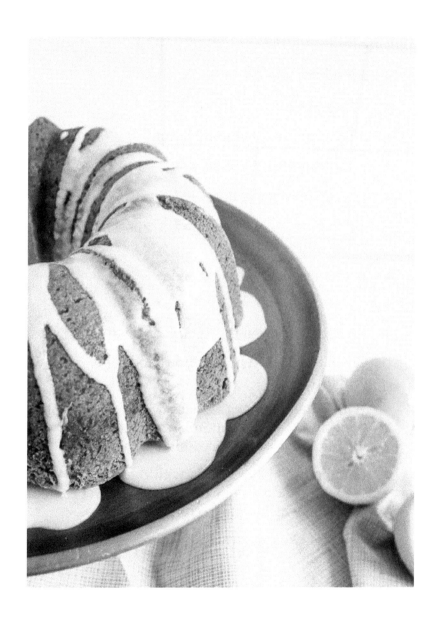

Preparation Time : 20 minutes

Cooking Time : 20minutes

Servings : 6

Ingredients :

- 2 Medium lemons
- 4 Large eggs
- 2 Tablespoons of almond butter
- 2 Tablespoons of avocado oil
- 1/3 cup of coconut flour
- 4-5 tablespoons of honey (or another sweetener of your choice)
- 1/2 tablespoon of baking soda

Directions :

1. Preheat your oven to a temperature of about 350 F.

2. Crack the eggs in a large bowl and set two egg whites aside.

3. Whisk the 2 whites of eggs with the egg yolks, the honey, the oil, the almond butter, the lemon zest and the juice and whisk very well together.

4. Combine the baking soda with the coconut flour and gradually add this dry mixture to the wet ingredients and keep whisking for a couple of minutes.

5. Beat the two eggs with a hand mixer and beat the egg into foam.

6. Add the white egg foam gradually to the mixture with a silicone spatula.

7. Transfer your obtained batter to tray covered with a baking paper.

8. Bake your cake for about 20 to 22 minutes.

9. Let the cake cool for 5 minutes; then slice your cake.

10. Serve and enjoy your delicious cake!

Nutrition : Calories: 164; Fat: 12g; Carbohydrates: 7.1; Fiber: 2.7g; Protein: 10.9g

Roasted Cumin Carrots

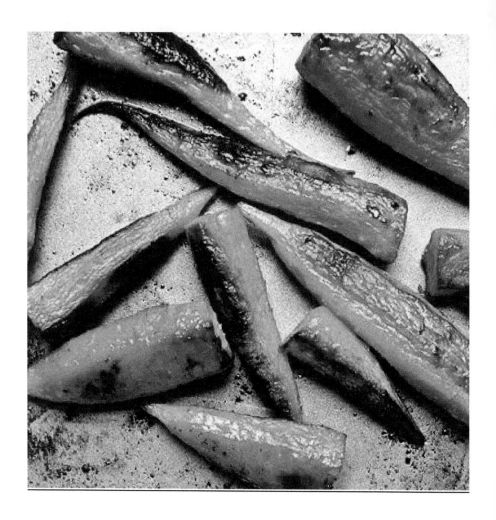

Preparation Time : 10 minutes

Cooking Time : 45 minutes

Servings : 4

Ingredients :

- 8 carrots, peeled and cut into 1/2-inch-thick slices
- 1 tsp. cumin seeds
- 1 tbsp. olive oil
- 1/2 tsp. kosher salt

Directions :

1. Preheat the oven to 400 F/ 200 C.
2. Line baking tray with parchment paper.
3. Add carrots, cumin seeds, olive oil, and salt in a large bowl and toss well to coat.
4. Spread carrots on a prepared baking tray and roast in preheated oven for 20 minutes.
5. Turn carrots to another side and roast for 20 minutes more.
6. Serve and enjoy.

Nutrition : Calories 82; Fat 3.6 g; Carbohydrates 12.2 g; Sugar 6 g; Protein 1.1 g; Cholesterol 0 mg

Tasty & Tender Brussels Sprouts

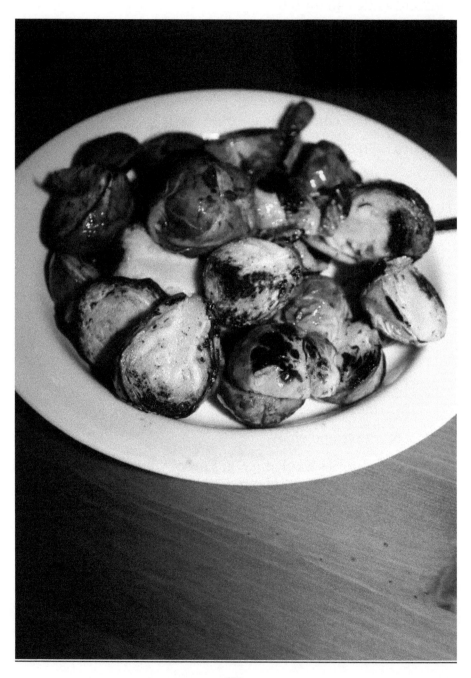

Preparation Time : 10 minutes

Cooking Time : 35 minutes

Servings : 4

Ingredients :

- 1 lb. Brussels sprouts, trimmed cut in half
- ¼ cup balsamic vinegar
- 1 onion, sliced
- 1 tbsp. olive oil

Directions :

1. Add water in a saucepan and bring to boil.
2. Add Brussels sprouts and cook over medium heat for 20 minutes. Drain well.
3. Heat oil in a pan over medium heat.
4. Add onion and cook until softened. Add sprouts and vinegar and stir well and cook for 1-2 minutes.
5. Serve and enjoy.

Nutrition : Calories 93; Fat 3.9 g; Carbohydrates 13 g; Sugar 3.7 g; Protein 4.2 g; Cholesterol 0 mg

Sautéed Veggies

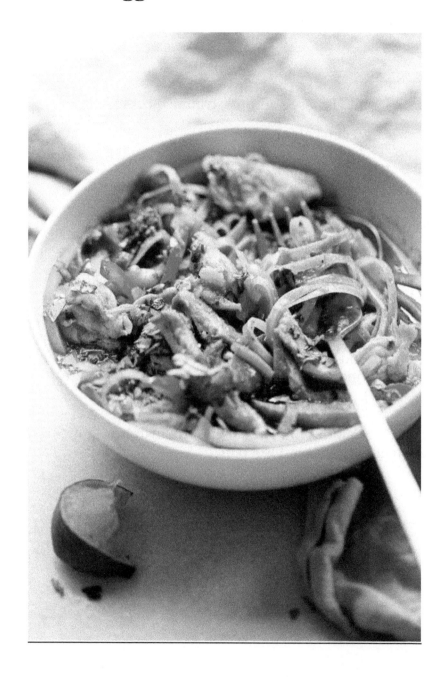

Preparation Time : 10 minutes

Cooking Time : 15 minutes

Servings : 4

Ingredients :

- 1/2 cup mushrooms, sliced
- 1 zucchini, diced
- 1 squash, diced
- 2 1/2 tsp. southwest seasoning
- 3 tbsp. olive oil

Directions :

1. In a medium bowl, whisk together southwest seasoning, pepper, olive oil, and salt.
2. Add vegetables to a bowl and mix well to coat.
3. Heat pan over medium-high heat.
4. Add vegetables in the pan and sauté for 5-7 minutes.
5. Serve and enjoy.

Nutrition : Calories 107; Fat 10.7 g; Carbohydrates 3.6 g; Sugar 1.5 g; Protein 1.2 g; Cholesterol 0 mg

Mustard Green Beans

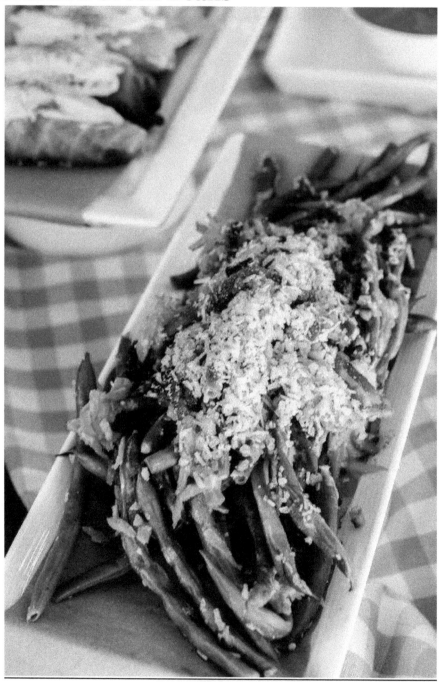

Preparation Time : 10 minutes

Cooking Time : 20 minutes

Servings : 4

Ingredients :

- 1 lb. green beans, washed and trimmed
- 1 tsp. whole grain mustard
- 1 tbsp. olive oil
- 2 tbsp. apple cider vinegar
- 1/4 cup onion, chopped

Directions :

1. Steam green beans in the microwave until tender.
2. Meanwhile, in a pan heat olive oil over medium heat.
3. Add the onion in a pan sauté until softened.
4. Add water, apple cider vinegar, and mustard in the pan and stir well.
5. Add green beans and stir to coat and heat through.
6. Season green beans with pepper and salt.
7. Serve and enjoy.

Nutrition : Calories 71; Fat 3.7 g; Carbohydrates 8.9 g; Sugar 1.9 g; Protein 2.1 g; Cholesterol 0 mg

Zucchini Fries

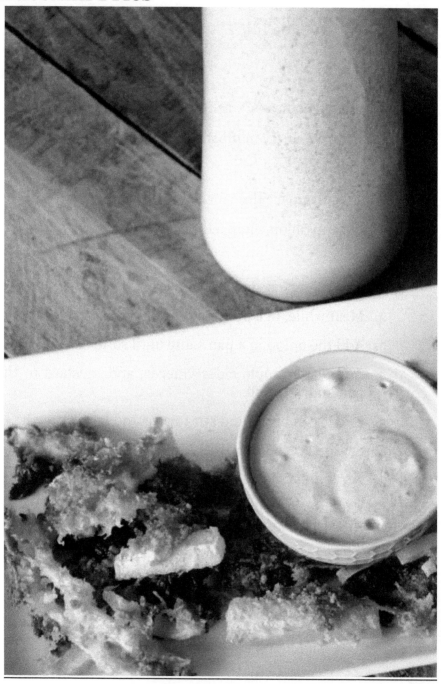

Preparation Time : 10 minutes

Cooking Time : 40 minutes

Servings : 4

Ingredients :

- 1 egg
- 2 medium zucchinis, cut into fry's shape
- 1 tsp. Italian herbs
- 1 tsp. garlic powder
- 1 cup parmesan cheese, grated

Directions :

1. Preheat the oven to 425 F/ 218 C.
2. Spray a baking tray with cooking spray and set aside.
3. In a small bowl, add egg and lightly whisk it.
4. In a separate bowl, mix together spices and parmesan cheese.
5. Dip zucchini fries in egg then coat with parmesan cheese mixture and place on a baking tray.
6. Bake in preheated oven for 25-30 minutes. Turn halfway through.
7. Serve and enjoy.

Nutrition : Calories 184; Fat 10.3 g; Carbohydrates 3.9 g; Sugar 2 g; Protein 14.7 g; Cholesterol 71 mg

Broccoli Nuggets

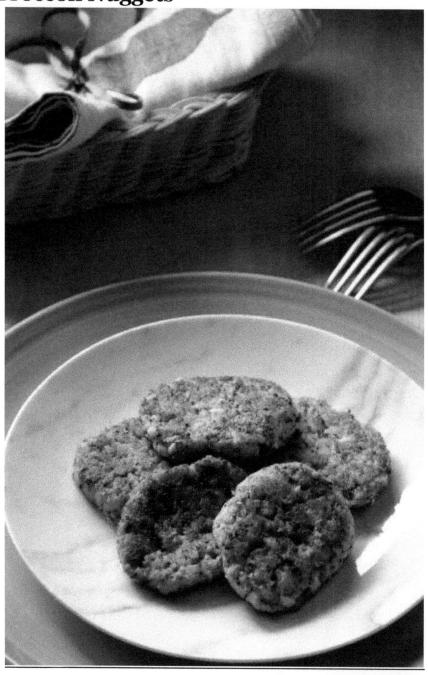

Preparation Time : 10 minutes

Cooking Time : 25 minutes

Servings : 4

Ingredients :

- 2 cups broccoli florets
- 1/4 cup almond flour
- 2 egg whites
- 1 cup cheddar cheese, shredded
- 1/8 tsp. salt

Directions :

1. Preheat the oven to 350 F/ 180 C.
2. Spray a baking tray with cooking spray and set aside.
3. Using potato masher breaks the broccoli florets into small pieces.
4. Add remaining ingredients to the broccoli and mix well.
5. Drop 20 scoops onto baking tray and press lightly into a nugget shape.
6. Bake in preheated oven for 20 minutes.
7. Serve and enjoy.

Nutrition : Calories 148; Fat 10.4 g; Carbohydrates 3.9 g; Sugar 1.1 g; Protein 10.5; Cholesterol 30 mg

Zucchini Cauliflower Fritters

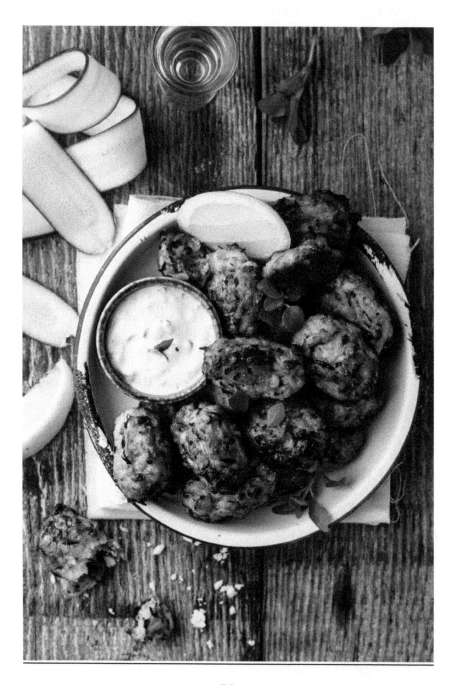

Preparation Time : 10 minutes

Cooking Time : 15 minutes

Servings : 4

Ingredients :

- 2 medium zucchinis, grated and squeezed
- 3 cups cauliflower florets
- 1 tbsp. coconut oil
- 1/4 cup coconut flour
- 1/2 tsp. sea salt

Directions :

1. Steam cauliflower florets for 5 minutes.
2. Add cauliflower into the food processor and process until it looks like rice.
3. Add all ingredients except coconut oil to the large bowl and mix until well combined.
4. Make small round patties from the mixture and set aside.
5. Heat coconut oil in a pan over medium heat.
6. Place patties in a pan and cook for 3-4 minutes on each side.
7. Serve and enjoy.

Nutrition : Calories 68 Fat 3.8 g; Carbohydrates 7.8 g; Sugar 3.6 g; Protein 2.8 g; Cholesterol 0 mg

Roasted Chickpeas

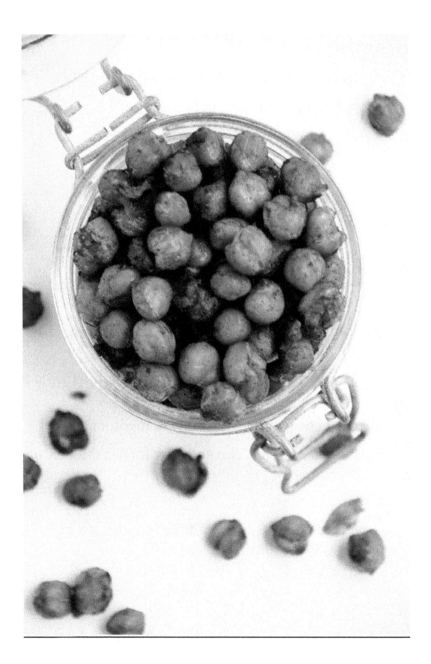

Preparation Time : 10 minutes

Cooking Time : 30 minutes

Servings : 4

Ingredients :

- 15 oz. can chickpeas, drained, rinsed and pat dry
- 1/2 tsp. paprika
- 1 tbsp. olive oil
- 1/2 tsp. pepper
- 1/2 tsp. salt

Directions :

1. Preheat the oven to 450 F/ 232 C.
2. Spray a baking tray with cooking spray and set aside.
3. In a large bowl, toss chickpeas with olive oil, paprika, pepper, and salt.
4. Spread chickpeas on a prepared baking tray and roast in preheated oven for 25 minutes. Stir every 10 minutes.
5. Serve and enjoy.

Nutrition : Calories 158; Fat 4.8 g; Carbohydrates 24.4 g; Sugar 0 g; Protein 5.3 g; Cholesterol 0 mg

Peanut Butter Mousse

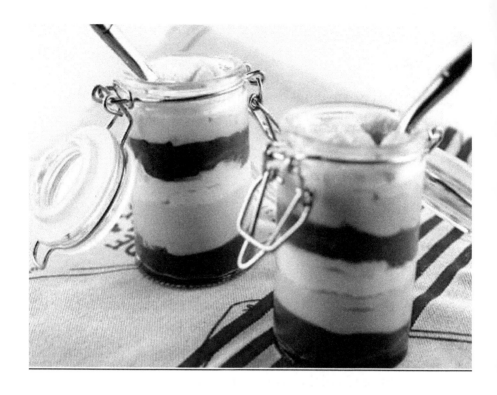

Preparation Time : 10 minutes

Cooking Time : 10 minutes

Servings : 2

Ingredients :

- 1 tbsp. peanut butter
- 1 tsp. vanilla extract
- 1 tsp. stevia
- 1/2 cup heavy cream

Directions :

1. Add all ingredients into the bowl and whisk until soft peak forms.
2. Spoon into the serving bowls and enjoy.

Nutrition : Calories 157; Fat 15.1 g; Carbohydrates 5.2 g; Sugar 3.6 g; Protein 2.6 g; Cholesterol 41 mg

Coffee Mousse

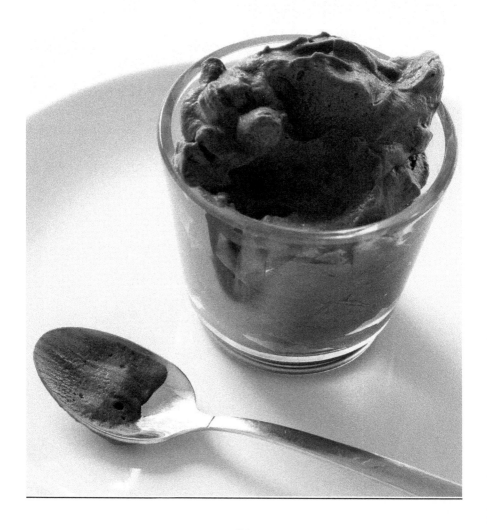

Preparation Time : 10 minutes

Cooking Time : 20 minutes

Servings : 8

Ingredients :

- 4 tbsp. brewed coffee
- 16 oz. cream cheese, softened
- 1/2 cup unsweetened almond milk
- 1 cup whipping cream
- 2 tsp. liquid stevia

Directions :

1. Add coffee and cream cheese in a blender and blend until smooth.
2. Add stevia, and milk and blend again until smooth.
3. Add cream and blend until thickened.
4. Pour into the serving glasses and place in the refrigerator.
5. Serve chilled and enjoy.

Nutrition : Calories 244; Fat 24.6 g; Carbohydrates 2.1 g; Sugar 0.1 g; Protein 4.7 g; Cholesterol 79 mg

Wild Rice and Black Lentils Bowl

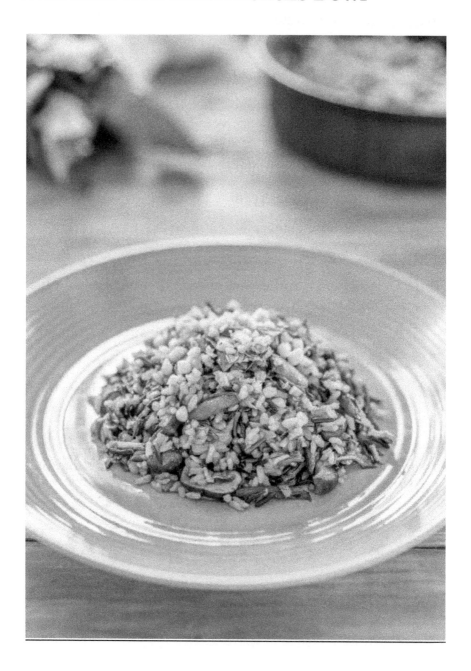

Preparation Time : 10 minutes

Cooking Time : 50 minutes

Servings : 4

Ingredients :

- Wild rice
- 2 cups wild rice, uncooked
- 4 cups spring water
- ½ teaspoon salt
- 2 bay leaves
- Black lentils
- 2 cups black lentils, cooked
- 1 ¾ cups coconut milk, unsweetened
- 2 cups vegetable stock
- 1 teaspoon dried thyme
- 1 teaspoon dried paprika
- ½ of medium purple onion; peeled, sliced
- 1 tablespoon minced garlic
- 2 teaspoons creole seasoning
- 1 tablespoon coconut oil
- Plantains
- 3 large plantains, chopped into ¼-inch-thick pieces
- 3 tablespoons coconut oil
- Brussels sprouts

- 10 large brussels sprouts, quartered

- 2 tablespoons spring water

- 1 teaspoon sea salt

- ½ teaspoon ground black pepper

Directions :

1. Prepare the rice: take a medium pot, place it over medium-high heat, pour in water, and add bay leaves and salt.

2. Bring the water to a boil, then switch heat to medium, add rice, and then cook for 30–45 minutes or more until tender.

3. When done, discard the bay leaves from rice, drain if any water remains in the pot, remove it from heat, and fluff by using a fork. Set aside until needed.

4. While the rice boils, prepare lentils: take a large pot, place it over medium-high heat and when hot, add onion and cook for 5 minutes or until translucent.

5. Stir garlic into the onion, cook for 2 minutes until fragrant and golden, then add remaining Ingredients for the lentils and stir until mixed.

6. Bring the lentils to a boil, then switch heat to medium and simmer the lentils for 20 minutes until tender, covering the pot with a lid.

7. When done, remove the pot from heat and set aside until needed.

8. While rice and lentils simmer, prepare the plantains: chop them into ¼-inch-thick pieces.

9. Take a large skillet pan, place it over medium heat, add coconut oil and when it melts, add half of the plantain pieces and cook for 7–10 minutes per side or more until golden-brown.

10. When done, transfer browned plantains to a plate lined with paper towels and repeat with the remaining plantain pieces; set aside until needed.

11. Prepare the sprouts: return the skillet pan over medium heat, add more oil if needed, and then add brussels sprouts.

12. Toss the sprouts until coated with oil, and then let them cook for 3–4 minutes per side until brown.

13. Drizzle water over sprouts, cover the pan with the lid, and then cook for 3–5 minutes until steamed.

14. Season the sprouts with salt and black pepper, toss until mixed, and transfer sprouts to a plate.

15. Assemble the bowl: divide rice evenly among four bowls and then top with lentils, plantain pieces, and sprouts.

16. Serve immediately.

Nutrition : Calories: 333; Carbohydrates: 49.2 g; Fat: 10.7 g; Protein: 6.2 g

Alkaline Spaghetti Squash Recipe

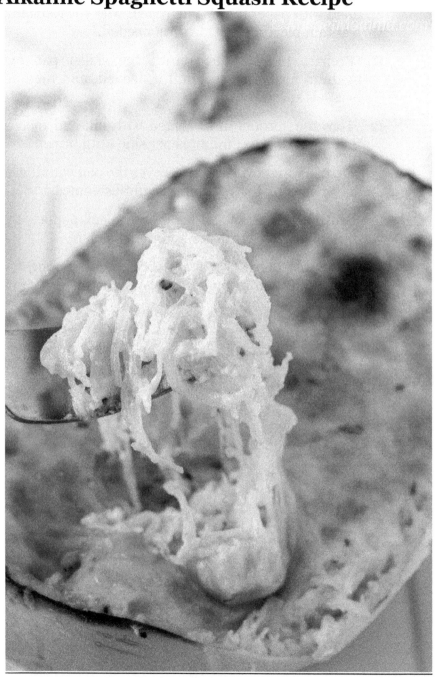

Preparation Time : 10 minutes

Cooking Time : 30 minutes

Servings : 4

Ingredients :

- 1 spaghetti squash
- Grapeseed oil
- Sea salt
- Cayenne powder (optional)
- Onion powder (optional)

Directions :

1. Preheat your oven to 375°f
2. Carefully chop off the ends of the squash and cut it in half.
3. Scoop out the seeds into a bowl.
4. Coat the squash with oil.
5. Season the squash and flip it over for the other side to get baked. When properly baked, the outside of the squash will be tender.
6. Allow the squash to cool off, then, use a fork to scrape the inside into a bowl.
7. Add seasoning to taste.
8. Dish your alkaline spaghetti squash!

Nutrition : Calories: 672; Carbohydrates: 65 g; Fat: 47 g; Protein: 12 g

Dairy-Free Fruit Tarts

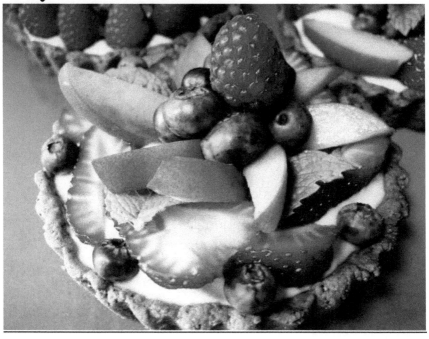

Preparation Time : 15 minutes

Cooking Time : 15 minutes

Servings : 2

Ingredients :

1 cup Coconut Whipped Cream

½ Easy Shortbread Crust (dairy-free option)

Fresh mint Sprigs

½ cup mixed fresh Berries

Directions :

1. Grease two 4" pans with detachable bottoms. Pour the shortbread mixture into pans and firmly press into the edges and bottom of each pan. Refrigerate for 15 minutes.

2. Loosen the crust carefully to remove from the pan.

3. Distribute the whipped cream between the tarts and evenly spread to the sides. Refrigerate for 1-2 hours to make it firm.

4. Use the berries and sprig of mint to garnish each of the tarts

Nutrition : Fat: 28.9g; Carbs: 8.3g; Protein: 5.8g; Calories: 306

Spaghetti Squash with Peanut Sauce

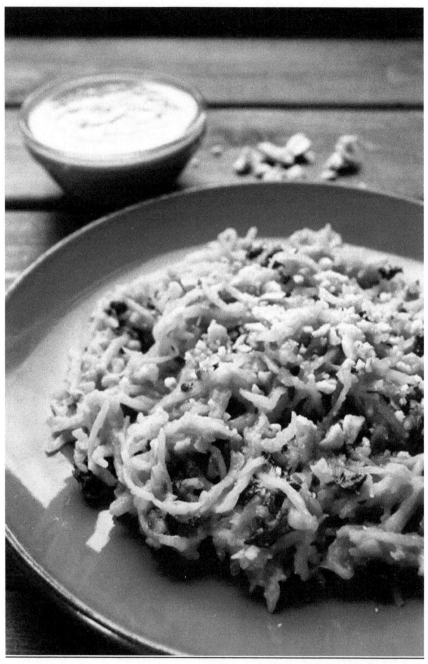

Preparation Time : 15 minutes

Cooking Time : 15 minutes

Servings : 4

Ingredients :

- 1 cup cooked shelled edamame; frozen, thawed
- 3-pound spaghetti squash
- ½ cup red bell pepper, sliced
- ¼ cup scallions, sliced
- 1 medium carrot, shredded
- 1 teaspoon minced garlic
- ½ teaspoon crushed red pepper
- 1 tablespoon rice vinegar
- ¼ cup coconut aminos
- 1 tablespoon maple syrup
- ½ cup peanut butter
- ¼ cup unsalted roasted peanuts, chopped
- ¼ cup and 2 tablespoons spring water, divided
- ¼ cup fresh cilantro, chopped
- 4 lime wedges

Directions :

1. Prepare the squash: cut each squash in half lengthwise and then remove seeds.

2. Take a microwave-proof dish, place squash halves in it cut-side-up, drizzle with 2 tablespoons water, and

then microwave at high heat setting for 10–15 minutes until tender.

3. Let squash cool for 15 minutes until able to handle. Use a fork to scrape its flesh lengthwise to make noodles, and then let noodles cool for 10 minutes.

4. While squash microwaves, prepare the sauce: take a medium bowl, add butter in it along with red pepper and garlic, pour in vinegar, coconut aminos, maple syrup, and water, and then whisk until smooth.

5. When the squash noodles have cooled, distribute them evenly among four bowls, top with scallions, carrots, bell pepper, and edamame beans, and then drizzle with prepared sauce.

6. Sprinkle cilantro and peanuts and serve each bowl with a lime wedge.

Nutrition : Calories: 419; Carbohydrates: 32.8 g; Fat: 24 g; Protein: 17.6 g

Cauliflower Alfredo Pasta

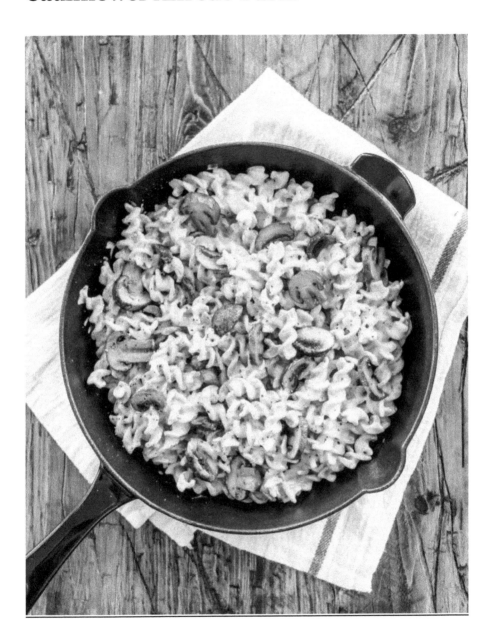

Preparation Time : 10 minutes

Cooking Time : 30 minutes

Servings : 4

Ingredients :

- Alfredo sauce
- 4 cups cauliflower florets, fresh
- 1 tablespoon minced garlic
- ¼ cup Nutritional yeast
- ½ teaspoon garlic powder
- ¾ teaspoon sea salt
- ½ teaspoon onion powder
- ½ teaspoon ground black pepper
- ½ tablespoon olive oil
- 1 tablespoon lemon juice, and more as needed for serving
- ½ cup almond milk, unsweetened
- Pasta
- 1 tablespoon minced parsley
- 1 lemon, juiced
- ½ teaspoon sea salt
- ¼ teaspoon ground black pepper
- 12 ounces spelt pasta; cooked, warmed

Directions :

1. Take a large pot half full with water, place it over medium-high heat, and then bring it to a boil.

2. Add cauliflower florets, cook for 10–15 minutes until tender, drain them well, and then return florets to the pot.

3. Take a medium skillet pan, place it over low heat, add oil and when hot, add garlic and cook for 4–5 minutes until fragrant and golden-brown.

4. Spoon garlic into a food processor, add remaining Ingredients for the sauce in it, along with cauliflower florets, and then pulse for 2–3 minutes until smooth.

5. Tip the sauce into the pot, stir it well, place it over medium-low heat, and then cook for 5 minutes until hot.

6. Add pasta into the pot, toss well until coated, taste to adjust seasoning, and then cook for 2 minutes until pasta gets hot.

7. Divide pasta and sauce among four plates, season with salt and black pepper, drizzle with lemon juice, and then top with minced parsley.

8. Serve straight away.

Nutrition : Calories: 360; Carbohydrates: 59 g; Fat: 9 g; Protein: 13 g

Sloppy Joe

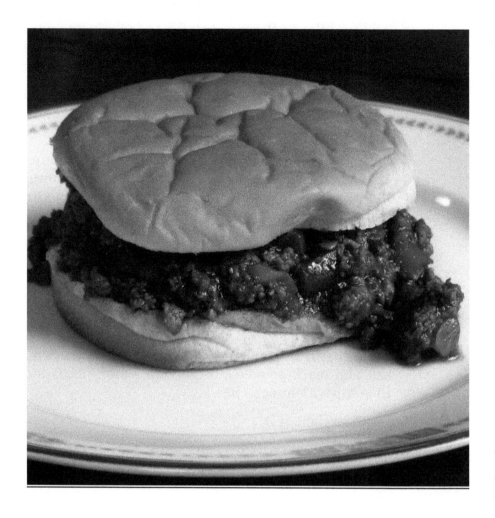

Preparation Time : 8 minutes

Cooking Time : 12 minutes

Servings : 4

Ingredients :

- 2 cups kamut or spelt wheat, cooked
- ½ cup white onion, diced
- 1 roma tomato, diced
- 1 cup chickpeas, cooked
- ½ cup green bell peppers, diced
- 1 teaspoon sea salt
- 1/8 teaspoon cayenne pepper
- 1 teaspoon onion powder
- 1 tablespoon grapeseed oil
- 1 ½ cups barbecue sauce, alkaline

Directions :

1. Plug in a high-power food processor, add chickpeas and spelt, cover with the lid, and then pulse for 15 seconds.

2. Take a large skillet pan, place it over medium-high heat, add oil and when hot, add onion and bell pepper, season with salt, cayenne pepper, and onion powder, and then stir until well combined.

3. Cook the vegetables for 3–5 minutes until tender. Add tomatoes, add the pulsed mixture, pour in barbecue sauce, and then stir until well mixed.

4. Simmer for 5 minutes, then remove the pan from heat and serve sloppy joe with alkaline flatbread.

Nutrition : Calories: 333; Carbohydrates: 65 g; Fat: 5 g; Protein: 14 g

Amaretti

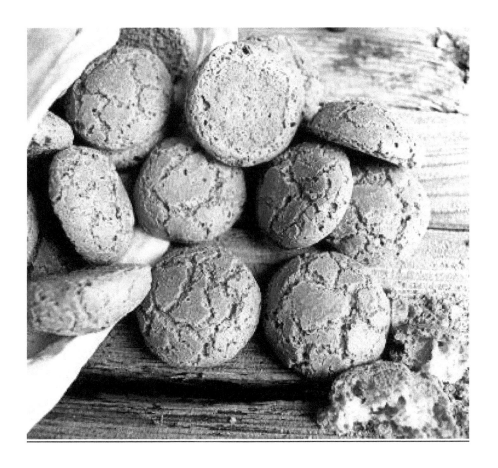

Preparation Time : 15 minutes

Cooking Time : 22 minutes

Servings : 2

Ingredients :

- ½ cup of granulated Erythritol-based Sweetener
- 165g (2 cups) sliced Almonds
- ¼ cup of powdered of Erythritol-based sweetener
- 4 large egg whites
- Pinch of salt
- ½ tsp. almond extract

Directions :

1. Heat the oven to 300° F and use parchment paper to line 2 baking sheets. Grease the parchment slightly.

2. Process the powdered sweetener, granulated sweetener, and sliced almonds in a food processor until it appears like coarse crumbs.

3. Beat the egg whites plus the salt and almond extracts using an electric mixer in a large bowl until they hold soft peaks. Fold in the almond mixture so that it becomes well combined.

4. Drop spoonful of the dough onto the prepared baking sheet and allow for a space of 1 inch between them. Press a sliced almond into the top of each cookie.

5. Bake in the oven for 22 minutes until the sides becomes brown. They will appear jellylike when they are taken out from the oven but will begin to be firms as it cools down.

Nutrition: Fat: 8.8g; Carbs: 4.1g; Protein: 5.3g; Calories: 117

Green Fruit Juice

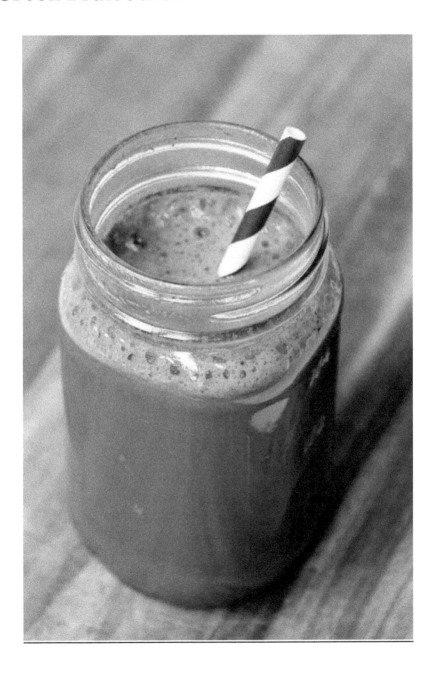

Preparation Time : 10 minutes

Cooking Time : 0 minutes

Servings : 2

Ingredients :

- 3 large kiwis, peeled and chopped
- 3 large green apples, cored and sliced
- 2 cups seedless green grapes
- 2 teaspoons fresh lime juice

Directions :

1. Add all ingredients into a juicer and extract the juice according to the manufacturer's method.
2. Pour into 2 glasses and serve immediately.

Nutrition : Calories 304; Total Fat 2.2 g; Saturated Fat 0 g; Protein 6.2 g

Kale Chickpea Mash

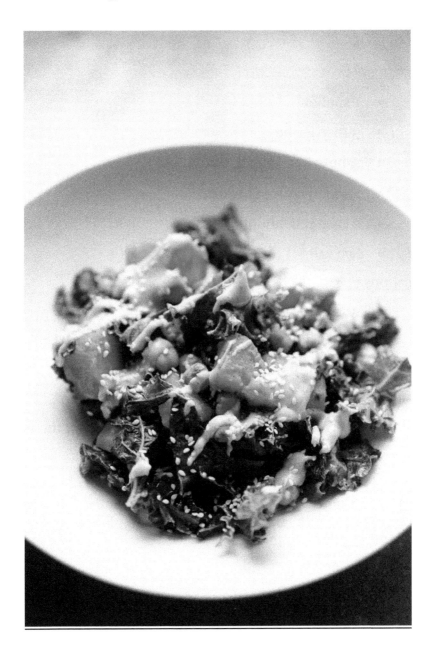

Preparation Time : 15 minutes

Cooking Time : 12 minutes

Servings : 1

Ingredients :

- 1 shallot
- 3 tbsp garlic
- A bunch of kale
- 1/2 cup boiled chickpea
- 2 tbsp coconut oil
- Sea salt

Directions :

1. Add some garlic in olive oil
2. Chop shallot and fry it with oil in a nonstick skillet.
3. Cook until the shallot turns golden brown.
4. Add kale and garlic in the skillet and stir well.
5. Add chickpeas and cook for 6 minutes. Add the rest of the Ingredients and give a good stir.
6. Serve and enjoy

Nutrition : Calories: 149; Total fat: 8 g; Saturated fat: 1 g; Net Carbohydrates: 13 g; Protein: 4 g; Sugars 6g; Fiber 3g; Sodium 226mg; Potassium 205mg

Quinoa and Apple

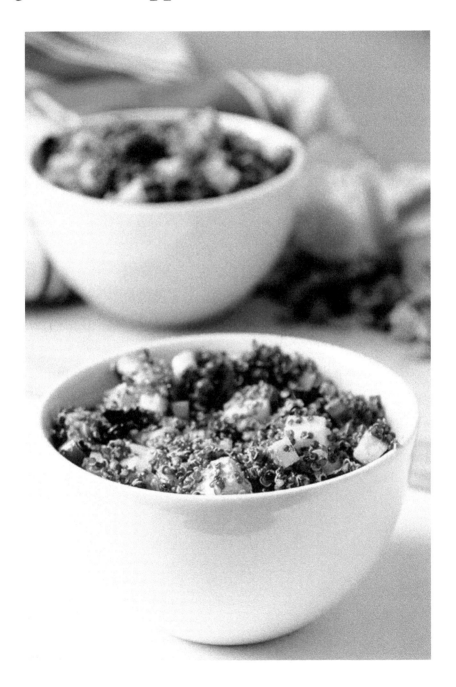

The combination of quinoa and apple yields a delicious and filling lunch dish that can be carried to work in your lunch box.

Preparation Time : 15 minutes

Cooking Time : 12 minutes

Servings : 1

Ingredients :

- 1/2 cup quinoa

- 1 apple

- 1/2 lemon

- Cinnamon to taste

Directions :

1. Cook quinoa according to the packet Directions.

2. Grate the apple and add to the cooked quinoa. Cook for 30 seconds.

3. Serve in a bowl then sprinkle lime and cinnamon. Enjoy.

Nutrition : Calories 229; Total fat: 3.2 g; Net Carbs: 32.3 g; Protein: 6.1 g; Sugars: 4.2 g; Fiber: 3.3 g; Sodium: 35.5 mg; Potassium: 211.8 mg